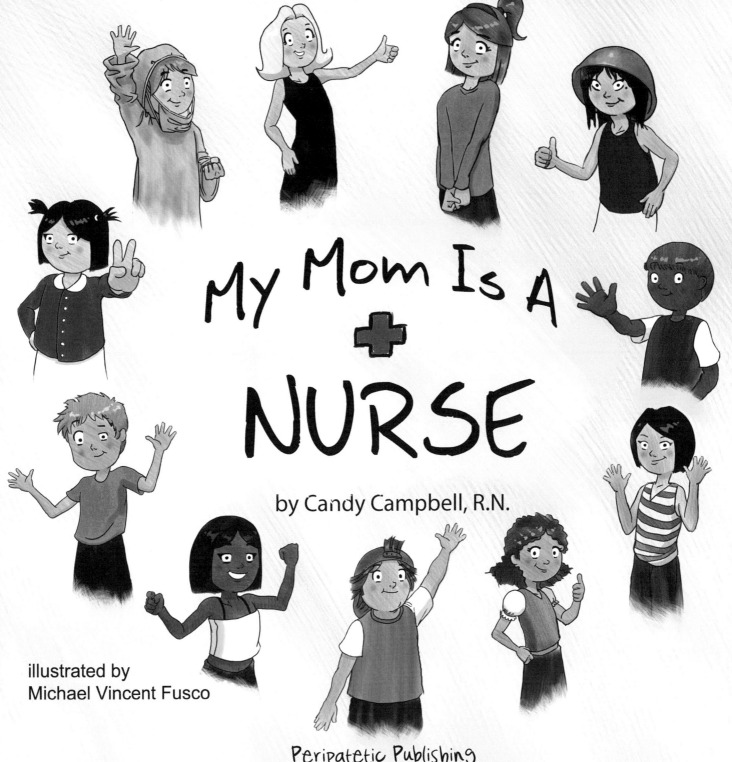

My Mom Is A ✚ NURSE

by Candy Campbell, R.N.

illustrated by
Michael Vincent Fusco

Peripatetic Publishing

My Mom is a Nurse/ by Candy Campbell; illustrated by Michael Vincent Fusco. -1st ed.

Summary: Children from many cultures are introduced to some of the important and exciting work that nurses do.

ISBN-13: 978-0-984238-50-7

Primary Category - Family and Relationship / Parenting / Motherhood

For information visit www.peripateticproductions.com

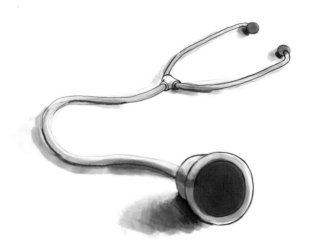

My mom is a nurse.
She cares for people.

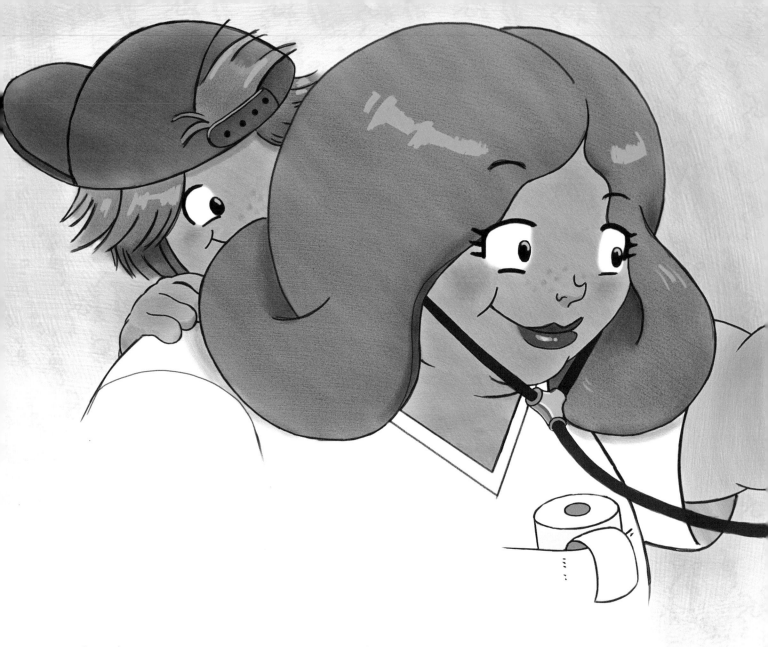

In the Emergency Room she puts a
bandage on the part that hurts.

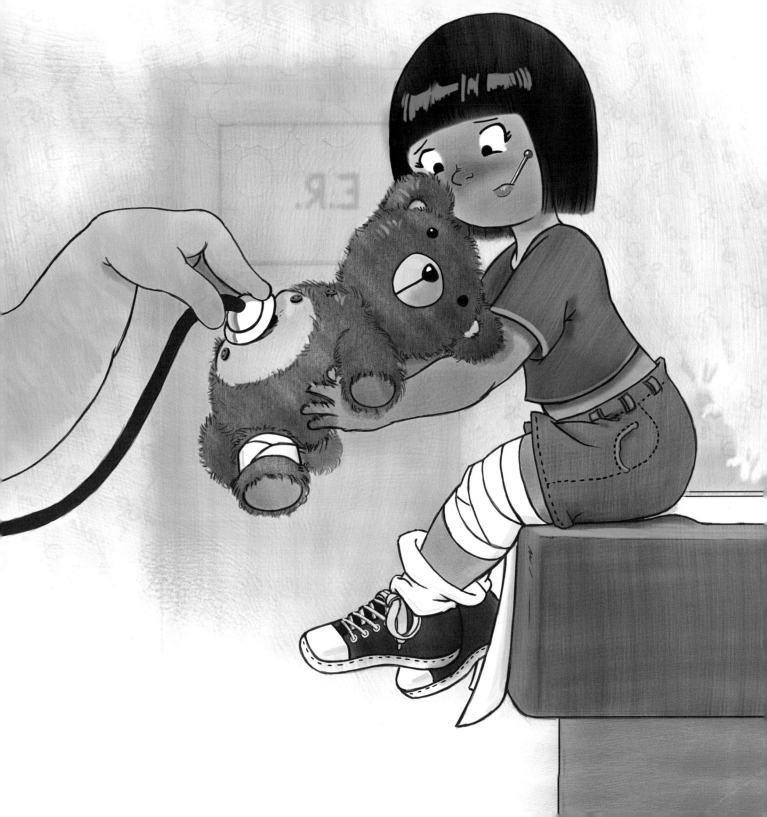

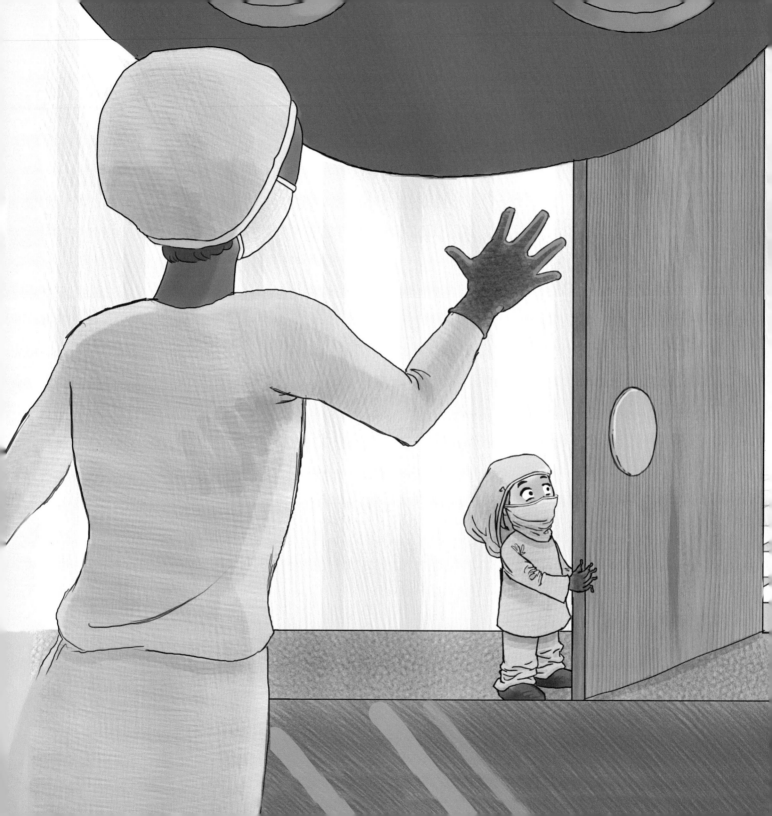

In the Operating Room she makes people feel better.

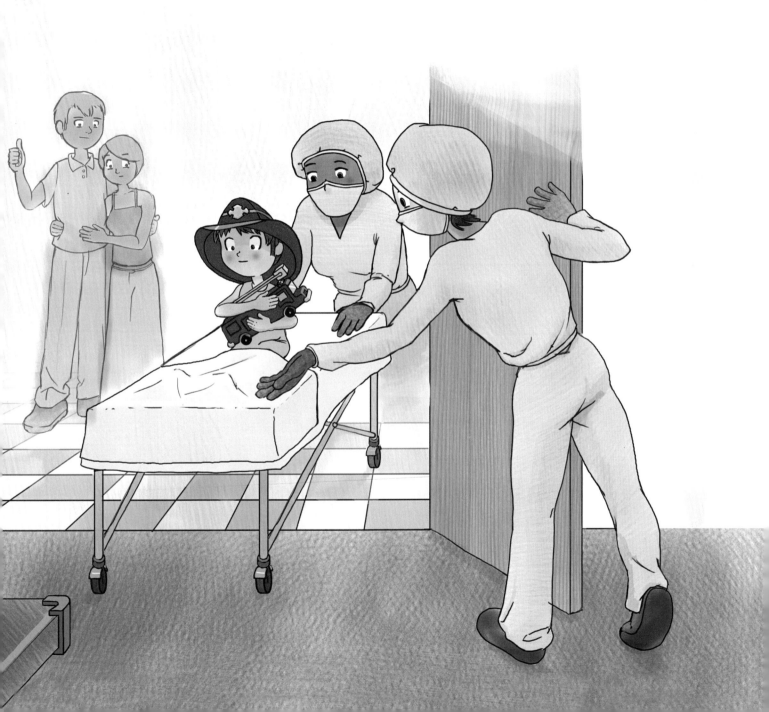

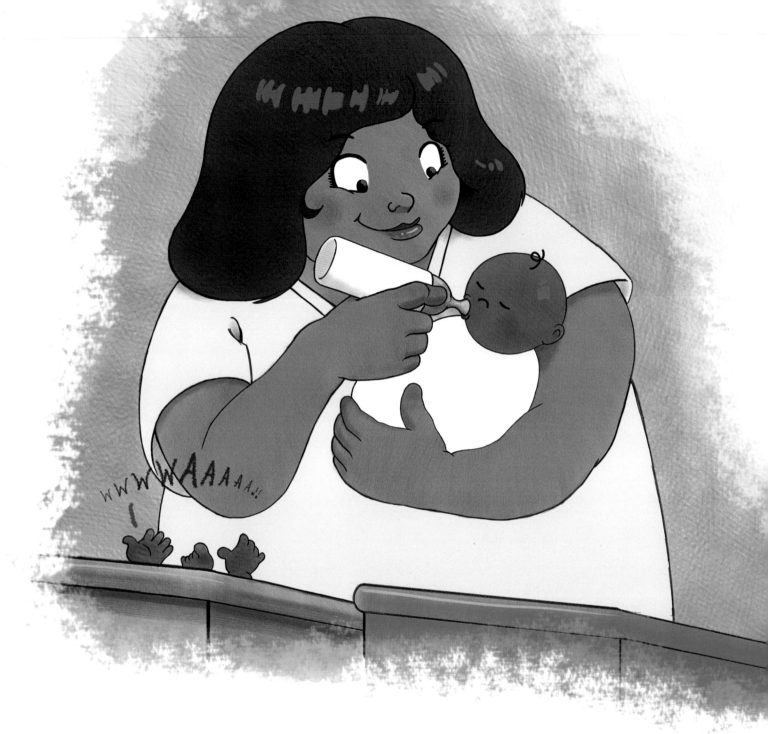

In the Nursery she takes care of sick babies.

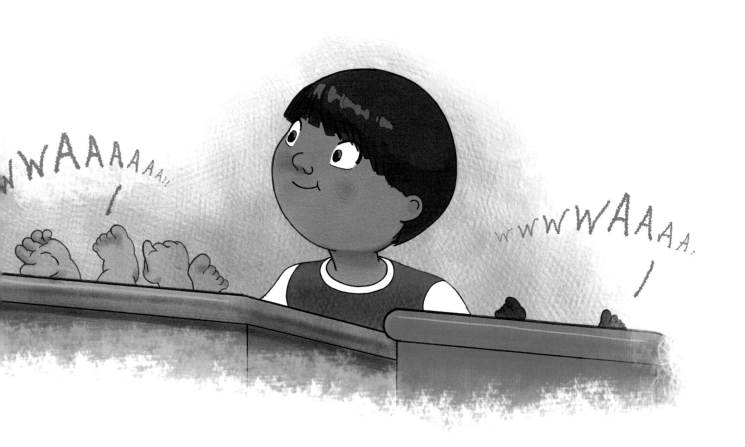

Sometimes she works in an ambulance.

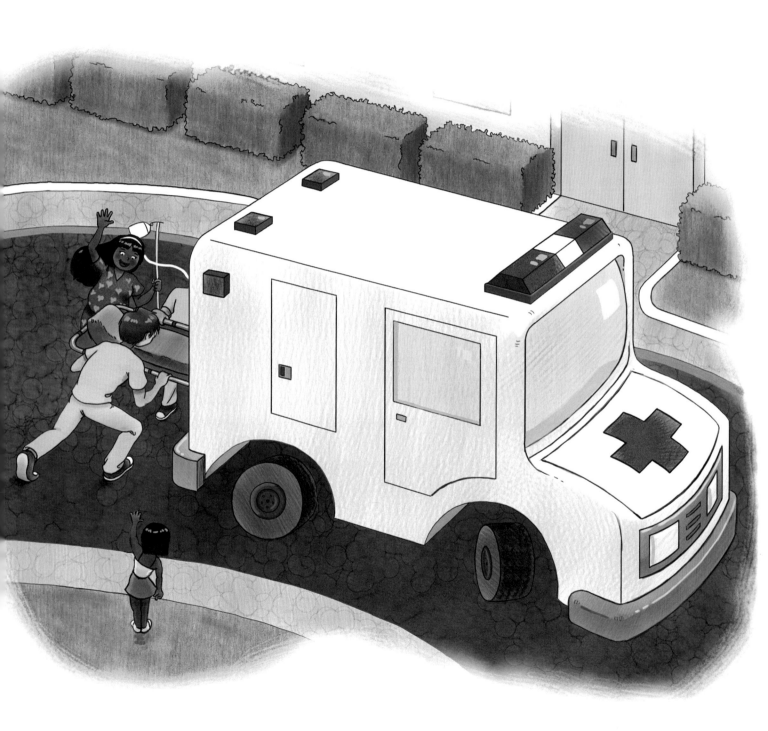

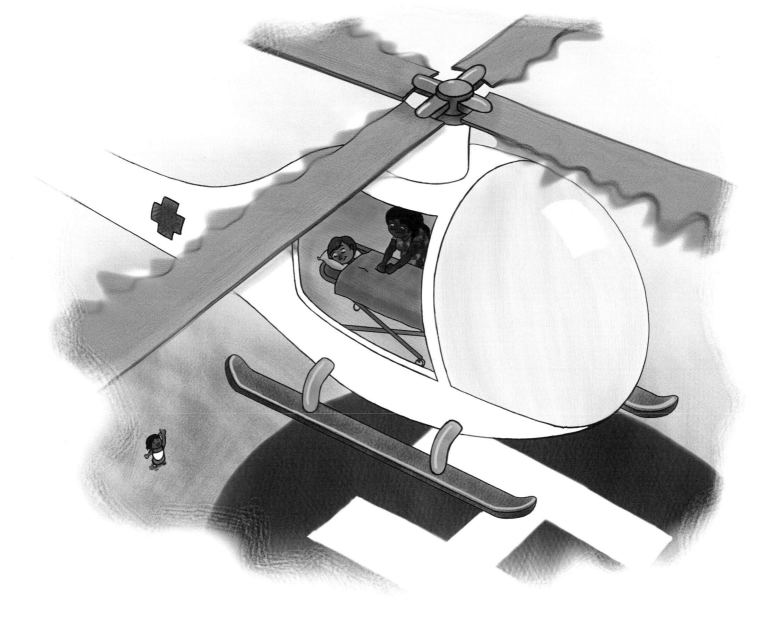

Sometimes she works in a helicopter.

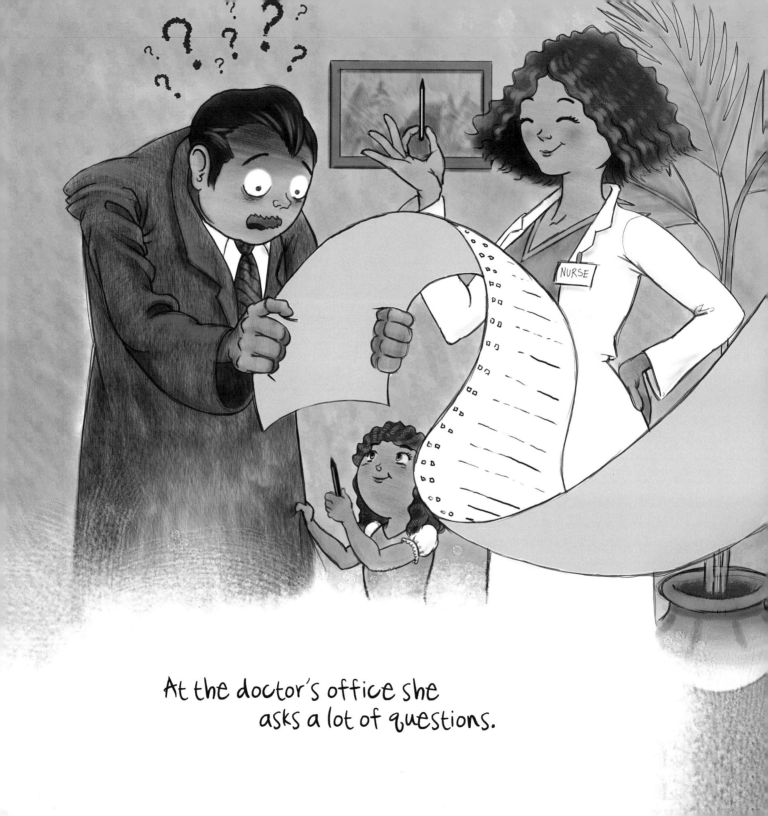

At the doctor's office she
asks a lot of questions.

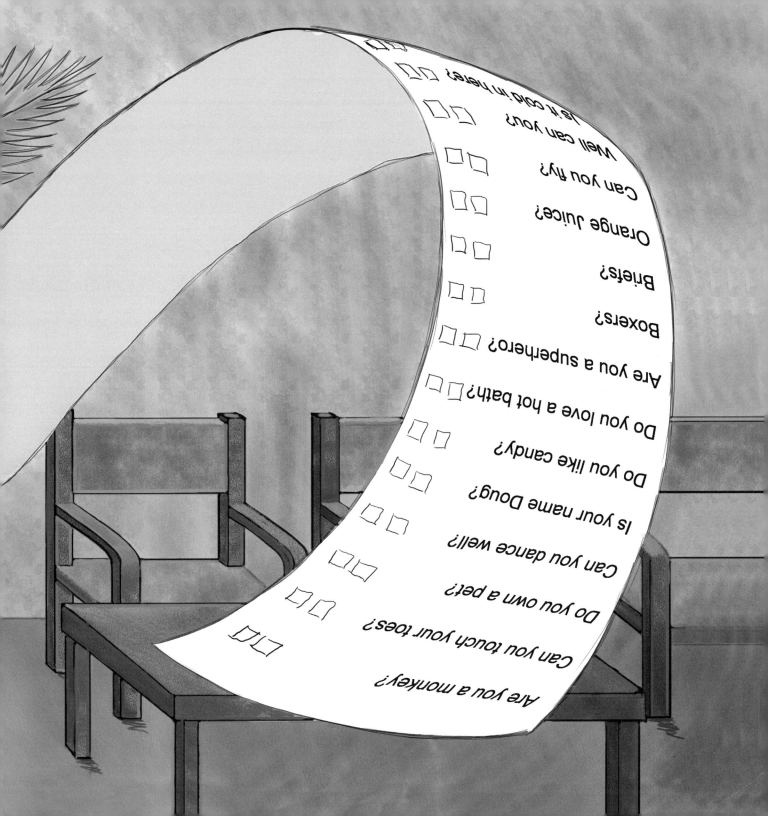

Come to think of it...

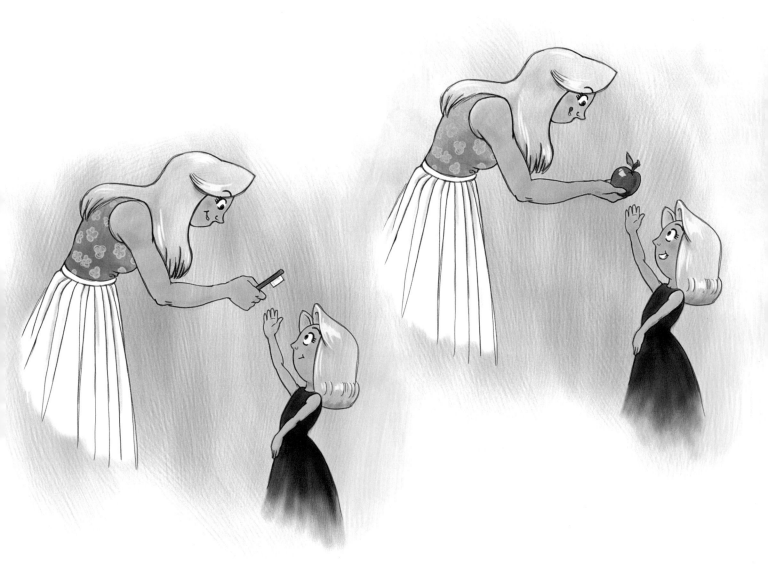

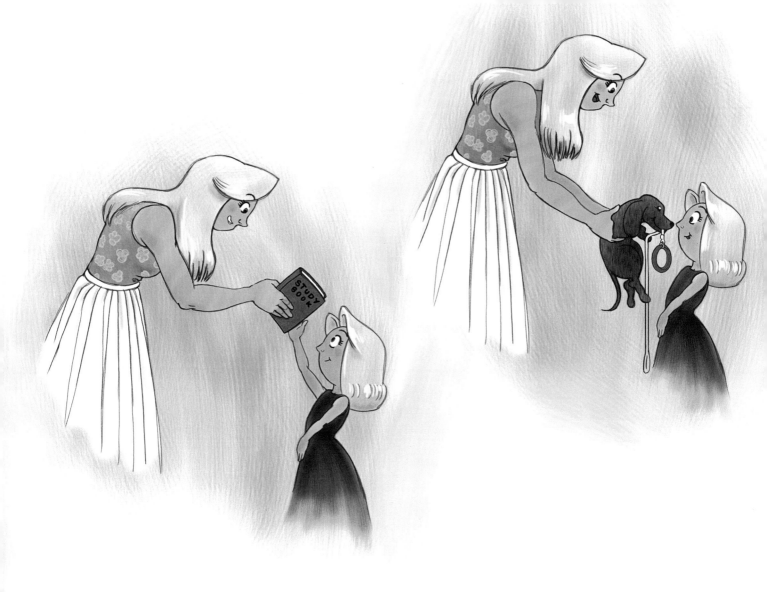

...she is always asking questions.

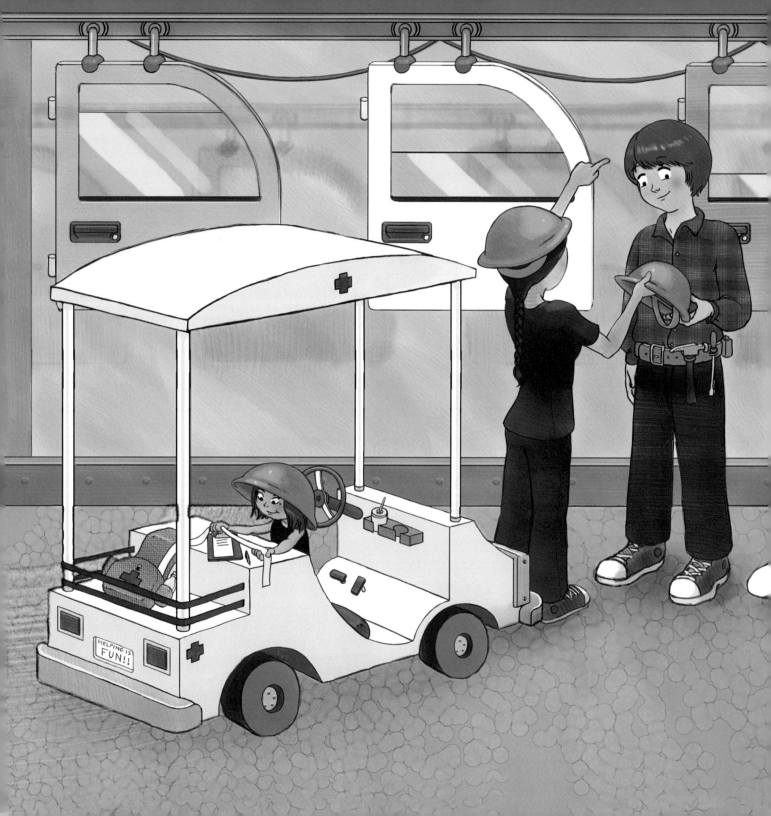

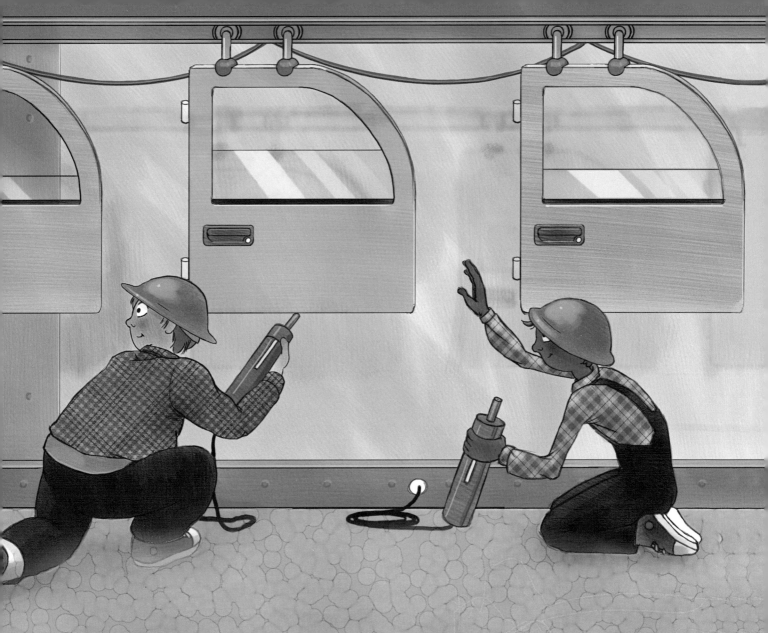

At the factory she helps keep people safe.

When she works at the school she teaches children how to take care of their bodies and stay healthy.

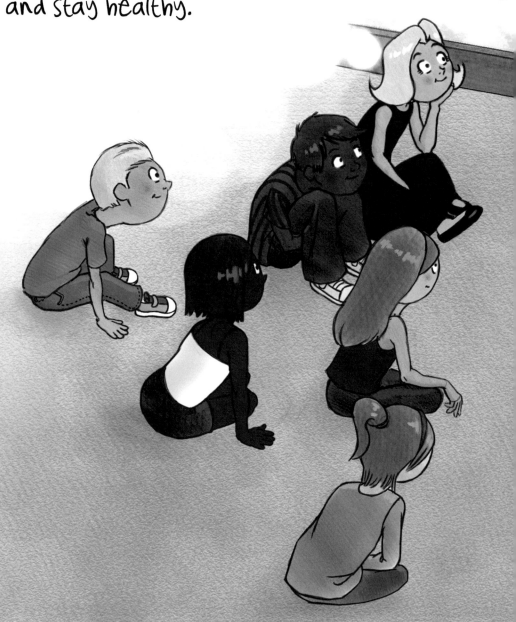

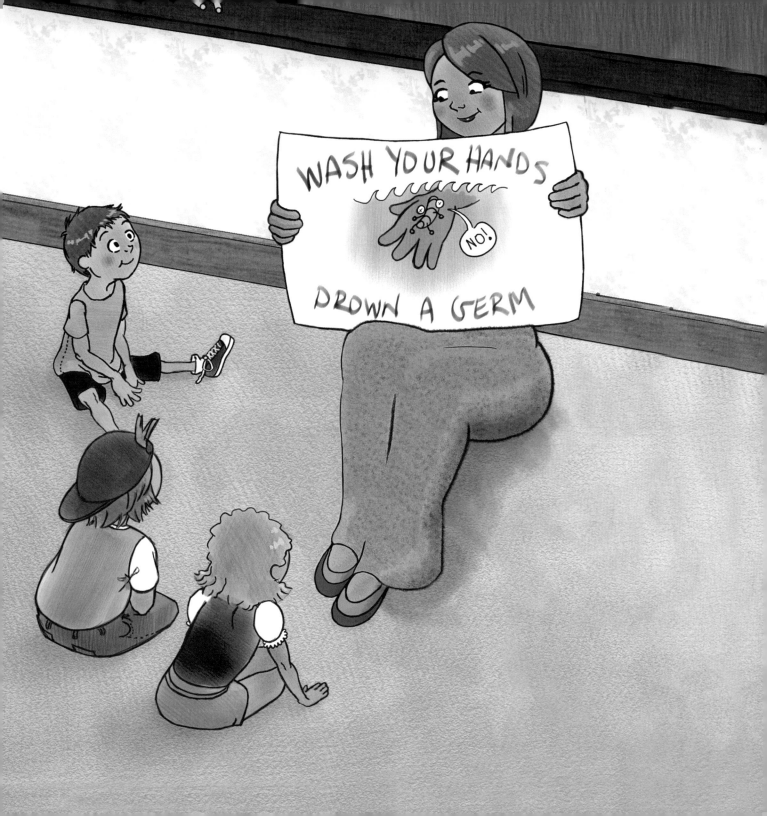

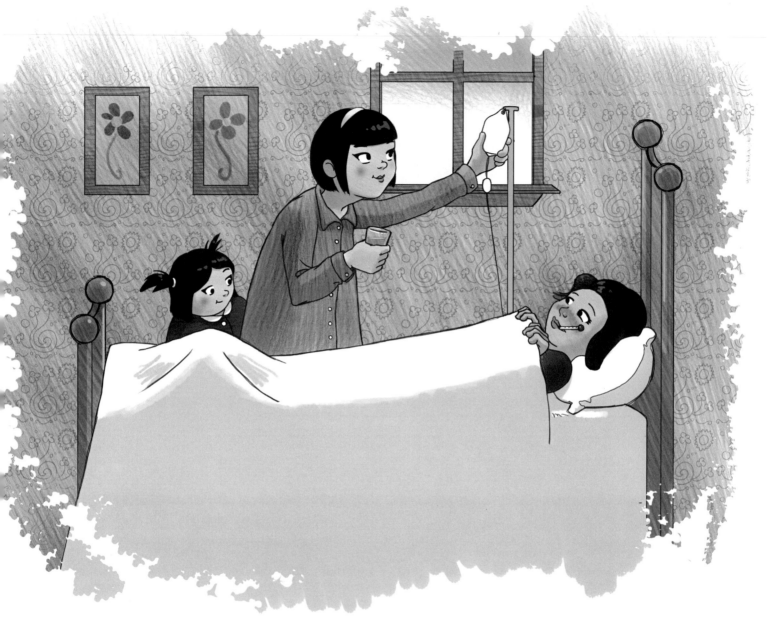

Sometimes she takes care of folks in their homes.

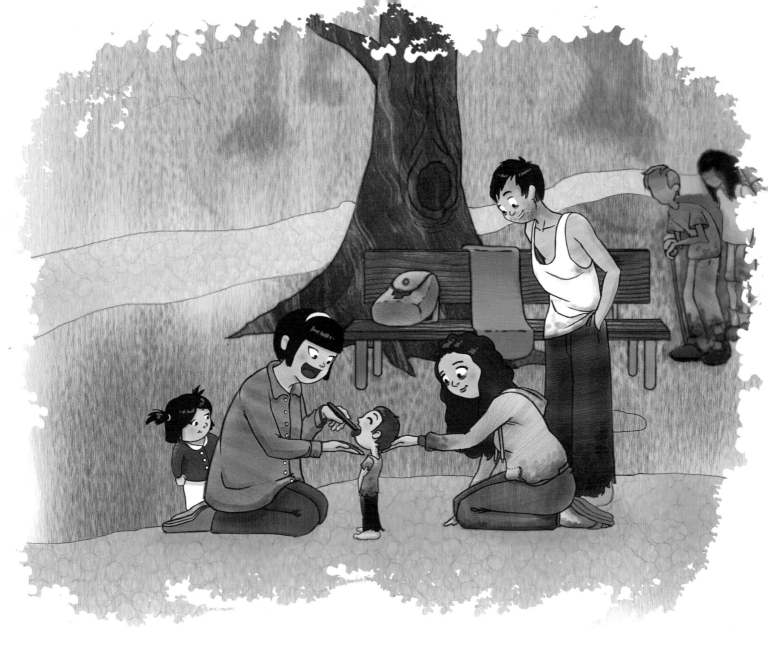

Sometimes she takes care of folks who have no home.

Sometimes she takes care of
soldiers hurt in battle.

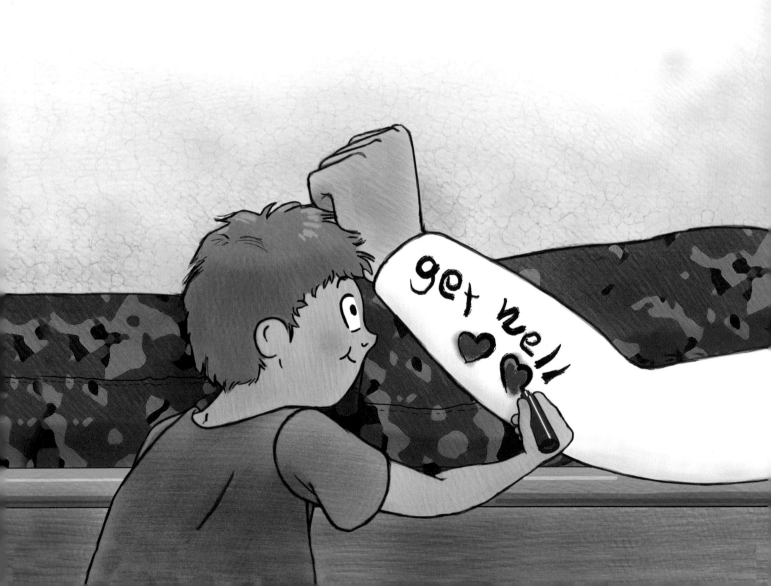

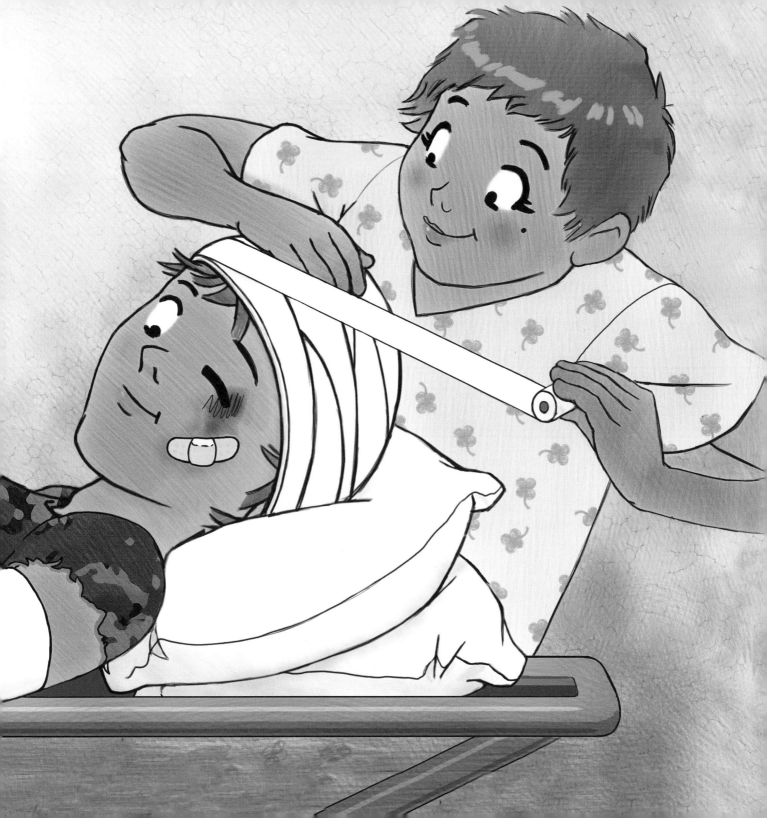

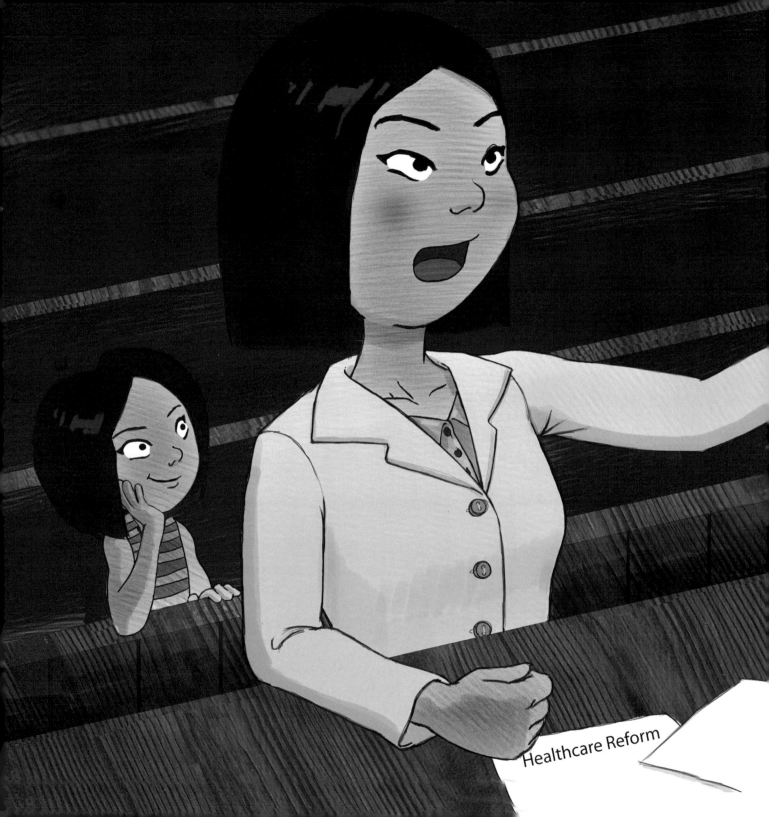

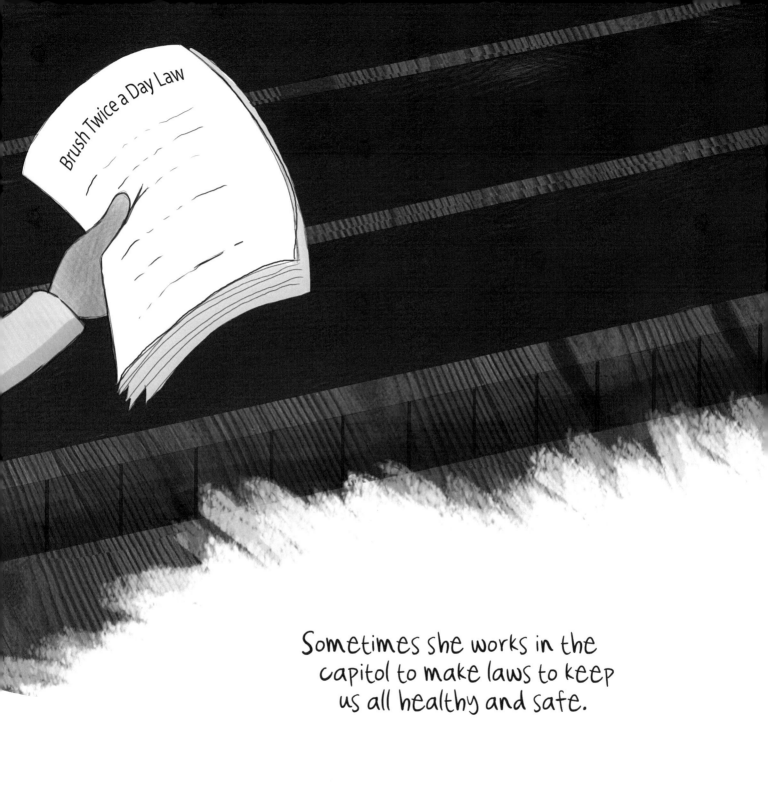

Sometimes she works in the capitol to make laws to keep us all healthy and safe.

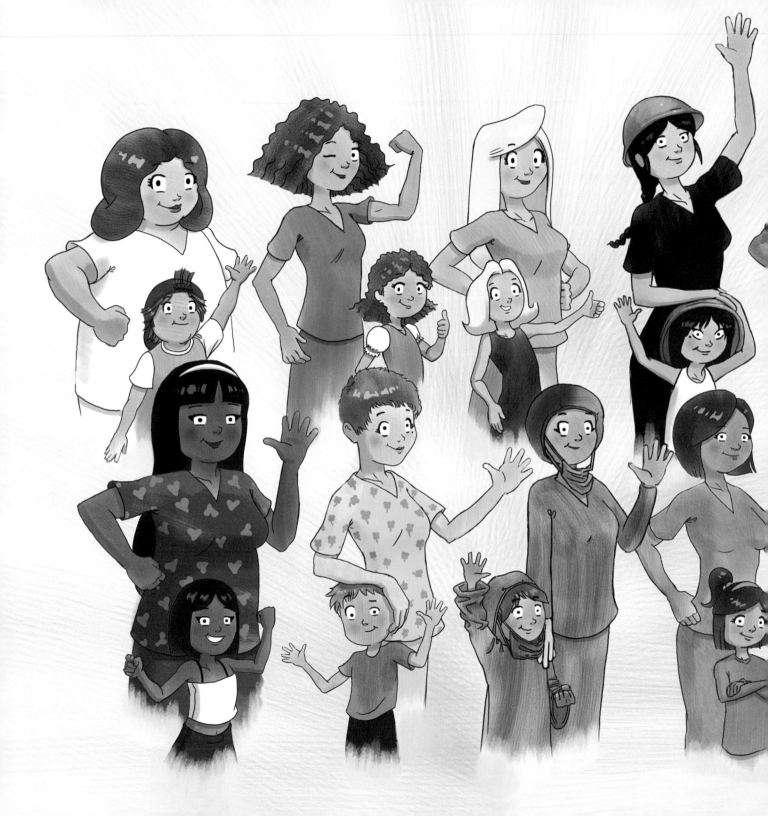

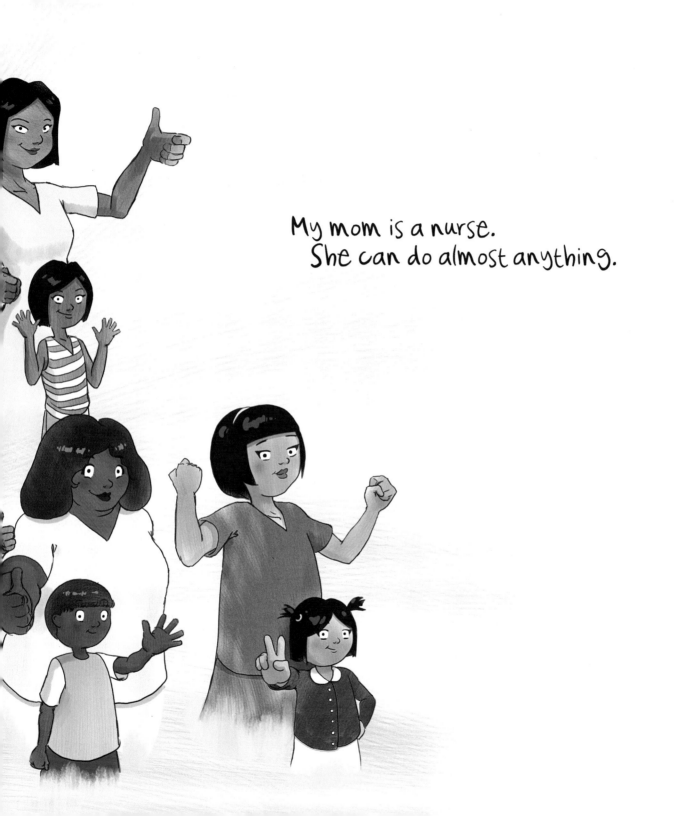

My mom is a nurse.
She can do almost anything.

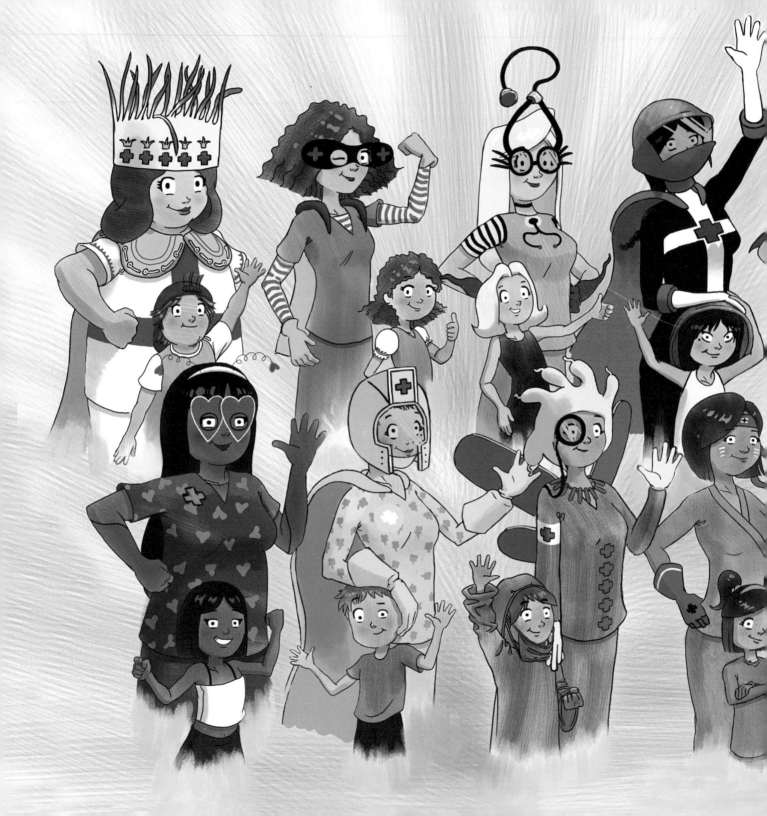

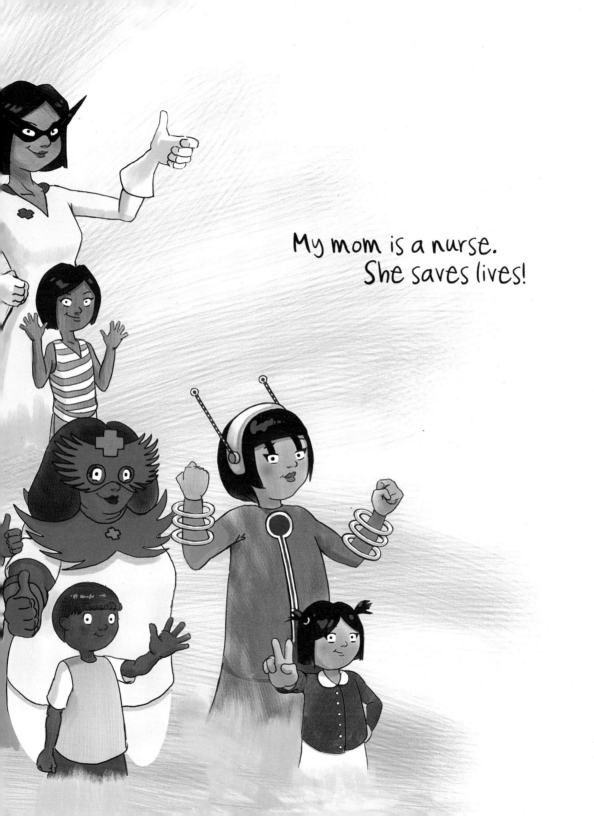

My mom is a nurse.
She saves lives!

Candy Campbell, R.N., resides in the San Francisco area where she spends her time as a nurse, a mom, a filmmaker, and an author. Look for the next children's book, *I Was a Premature Baby*, coming soon. Visit www.candycampbell.com for more info.

Michael Vincent Fusco resides in southern California where he illustrates children's books, creates fine art, designs clothing, and writes music. Examples of his work can be found at www.michaelvincentfuscoillustration.com.

CPSIA information can be obtained
at www.ICGtesting.com
Printed in the USA
LVRC02n0757300818
588492LV00001BE/5

* 9 7 8 0 9 8 4 2 3 8 5 0 7 *